PLANT BASED

DIET COOKBOOK

For Crohn's Colitis

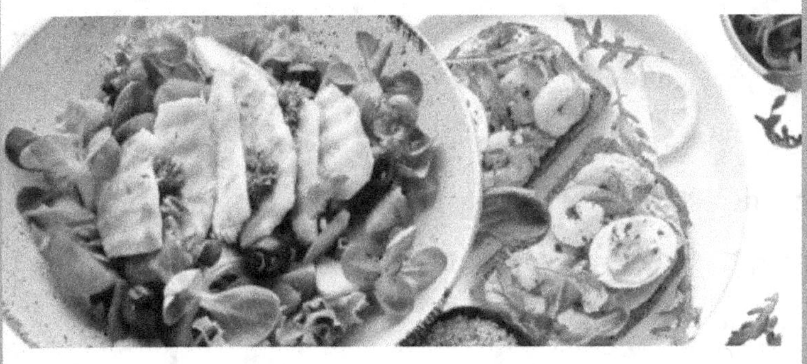

Healthy Delicious Recipes To Improve

Digestion And Relieve Inflammation

Leona Butler

Copyright © 2024 by LEONA BUTLER

This book is a work of fiction. Any references to historical events, real people, or real locales are

used fictitiously. Other names, characters, places, and incidents are products of the author's imagination, and any resemblance to actual events or locales or persons, living or dead, is entirely coincidental

Plant based diet cookbook for Crohn's and colitis

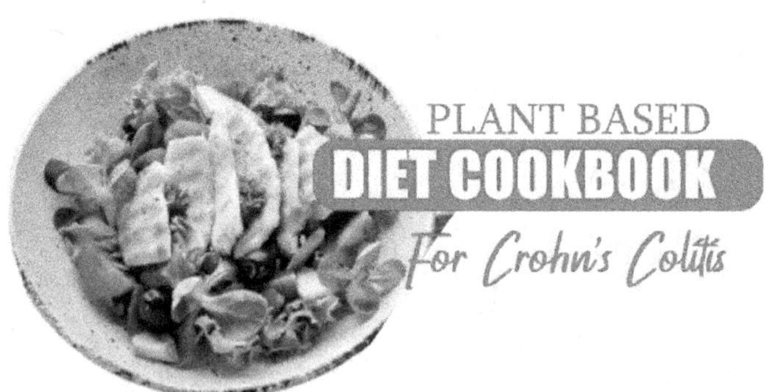

1. This Reliable Cookbook: Choose a plant-based cookbook specifically tailored for individuals with Crohn's and colitis. Look for authors or contributors with expertise in digestive health.

2. Read Introduction and Guidelines: Start by thoroughly reading the cookbook's introduction. Many provide helpful guidelines and insights on adapting a plant-based diet to manage Crohn's and colitis.

3. Familiarize Yourself with Ingredients: Take time to understand the recommended ingredients. Look for foods that are gentle on the digestive system and avoid those known to trigger symptoms.

4. Plan Balanced Meals: Use the cookbook to plan well-balanced meals. Ensure you incorporate a variety of fruits, vegetables, whole grains, and plant-based proteins to meet your nutritional needs.

5. Experiment with Recipes: Begin experimenting with simple recipes first. Pay attention to how your body reacts to different ingredients and make note of any triggers or improvements.

6. Modify Recipes if Necessary: Don't hesitate to modify recipes based on your personal tolerances. Adjust spice levels, cooking methods, or ingredient quantities to suit your digestive comfort.

7. Keep a Food Diary: Maintain a food diary to track what you eat and how it affects your symptoms. This can help identify patterns and guide future meal planning.

8. Consult with a Nutritionist: If possible, consult with a nutritionist familiar with managing Crohn's and colitis. They can provide personalized advice and help you optimize your plant-based diet.

Table Of Content

35 Delicious and Nutritious Plant based diet cookbook for Crohn's and colitis

Abstract

Discover a transformative culinary journey with our Plant-Based Diet Cookbook tailored for individuals managing Crohn's and colitis. This comprehensive guide features flavorful, gut-friendly recipes meticulously crafted to alleviate symptoms and promote digestive health.

Immerse yourself in a fusion of vibrant plant-based ingredients, skillfully curated to soothe inflammation and enhance nutrient absorption. From nourishing breakfasts to satisfying dinners, each recipe is thoughtfully designed to support gastrointestinal wellness.

Embrace a delicious path to healing, empowering individuals with Crohn's and colitis to thrive on a plant-based diet, fostering a harmonious relationship between nutrition and digestive well-being. Elevate your health through the artful and nutritious world of plant-based cuisine.

Introduction

Steven, once burdened by the relentless grip of Crohn's and colitis, discovered a transformative journey through dietary changes. Frustrated by conventional treatments, he delved into research, uncovering the impact of nutrition on gut health.

Embracing a holistic approach, Steven eliminated trigger foods, prioritizing anti-inflammatory options like leafy greens, lean proteins, and probiotic-rich foods. Slowly, his symptoms waned, replaced by a newfound vitality. Encouraged, Steven engaged in regular exercise, further enhancing his well-being.

The right diet became his shield against the debilitating effects of Crohn's and colitis. Steven's triumph inspired others, demonstrating the power of personalized nutrition in managing these conditions. His story exemplifies the potential for transformative change when armed with knowledge and a commitment to holistic health.

1. Vegan Pancakes Mk:

Ingredients:

- 1 cup all-purpose flour
- 1 tablespoon sugar
- 1 tablespoon baking powder
- 1/4 teaspoon salt
- cup plant-based milk
- tablespoons vegetable oil
- 1 teaspoon vanilla extract

Preparation:

1. In a bowl, combine the flour, sugar, baking powder, and salt.
2. Add plant-based milk, vegetable oil, and vanilla extract. Mix until just combined.
3. Heat a non-stick pan over medium heat and ladle batter onto the surface.
4. Cook until bubbles appear on the surface, then flip and cook the opposite side.

5. Serve with your favorite vegan toppings.

Nutritional Value (per serving):

- Calories: ~200

- Protein: ~5g

- Fat: ~8g

- Carbohydrates: ~28g

- Fiber: ~1g

Cooking Time:

Approximately 15 minutes.

2. Banana and Apple Pancakes:

Ingredients:

- 1 cup whole wheat flour

- 1 tablespoon sugar

- 1 tablespoon baking powder

- 1/4 teaspoon salt

- 1 ripe banana, mashed

- 1 apple, finely chopped

- cup almond milk

- tablespoons melted coconut oil

Preparation:

Combine whole wheat flour, sugar, baking powder, and salt in a bowl.

Add mashed banana, chopped apple, almond milk, and melted coconut oil. Mix until well combined.

Heat a pan over medium heat, spoon batter onto the surface, and cook until golden on both sides.

Top with fresh fruit or maple syrup.

Nutritional Value (per serving):

- Calories: ~250
- Protein: ~6g
- Fat: ~10g
- Carbohydrates: ~35g
- Fiber: ~4g

Cooking Time:

Approximately 20 minutes.

3. Banana, Blueberry, and Kale Smoothie

Ingredients:

- 1 ripe banana
- 1/2 cup blueberries (fresh or frozen)
- 1 cup chopped kale leaves, stems removed
- 1/2 cup Greek yogurt
- 1 cup almond milk (or your chosen milk)
- 1 tablespoon honey or maple syrup (optional) Ice cubes (optional)

Preparation:

1. Peel and slice the banana.
2. In a blender, combine banana slices, blueberries, chopped kale, Greek yogurt, almond milk, and honey (if using).
3. Blend until smooth and creamy.
4. If desired, add ice cubes and blend again to create a refreshing cold.

Nutritional Value:

- Calories: Approximately 250

- Protein: 10g

- Fiber: 8g

- Vitamins and minerals from kale, banana, and blueberries. Cooking Time:

5 minutes

Now, moving on to the Yogurt Parfait With Mixed Berries.

4. Yogurt Parfait With Mixed Berries

Ingredients:

- 1 cup Greek yogurt

- 1/2 cup granola

- 1/2 cup mixed berries (strawberries, blueberries, raspberries)

- 1 tablespoon honey or agave syrup 1 tablespoon chopped nuts (almonds, walnuts)

Preparation:

1. In a glass or bowl, place half of the Greek yogurt.

2. Add a layer of granola, followed by a layer of mixed berries.

3. Drizzle with honey or agave syrup.

4. Repeat the layers, finishing with a sprinkle of chopped nuts on top.

Nutritional Value:

- Calories: Approximately 300

- Protein: 15g

- Fiber: 6g

- Rich in probiotics, vitamins, and antioxidants from yogurt and berries.

Assembly Time:

5 minutes

Enjoy these nutritious and delicious smoothie and parfait recipes!

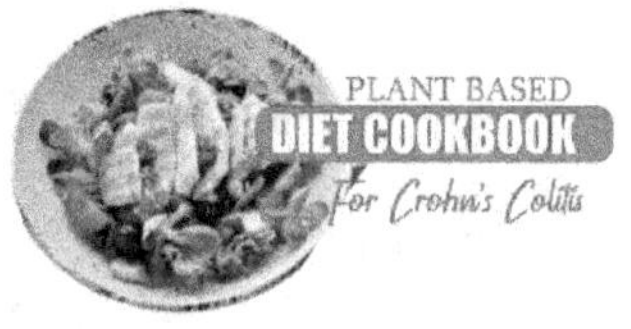

5. Overnight Oats

Ingredients:

- 1/2 cup rolled oats
- 1/2 cup milk (dairy or plant-based)
- 1/2 cup Greek yogurt
- 1 tablespoon chia seeds
- 1 tablespoon honey or maple syrup
- 1/2 teaspoon vanilla extract
- Fresh fruits (e.g., berries, banana slices) for topping

Preparation:

1. In a jar or container, combine rolled oats, milk, Greek yogurt, chia seeds, honey or maple syrup, and vanilla extract.
2. Stir thoroughly until all components are uniformly distributed.
3. Cover the jar or container and refrigerate overnight or for at least 4 hours.
4. Before serving, give it a good stir and top with fresh fruits.

Nutritional Value:

- Approximate calories: 350
- Protein: 15g
- Fiber: 8g
- Healthy fats: 8g

Cooking Time:

No cooking required, but refrigerate for at least 4 hours or overnight. Now, for Eggs, Salmon, and Avocado:

6. Eggs, Salmon, and Avocado

Ingredients:

- 2 eggs
- 4 oz smoked salmon
- 1 ripe avocado, sliced
- Salt and pepper to taste
- Optional: Fresh herbs (e.g., dill, chives) for garnish

Preparation:

1. Poach or fry the eggs to your liking.

2. Arrange the smoked salmon on a plate.

3. Place the poached or fried eggs on top of the salmon.

4. Add sliced avocado on the side.

5. Season with salt and pepper, and garnish with fresh herbs if desired.

Nutritional Value:

- Approximate calories: 450
- Protein: 25g
- Healthy fats: 30g
- Omega-3 fatty acids from salmon.

Cooking Time:

Eggs: 3-5 minutes depending on cooking method. No cooking required for salmon and avocado.

7. Baked Apple

Ingredients:

- 4 medium-sized apples

- 1/4 cup brown sugar

- teaspoon ground cinnamon

- tablespoons unsalted butter 1/2 cup chopped nuts (optional)

Preparation:

- Preheat the oven to 375°F (190°C).

- Core the apples, leaving the bottom intact, creating a well for the filling.

- In a small bowl, mix brown sugar and cinnamon.

- Stuff each apple with the sugar-cinnamon mixture. Place a small piece of butter on top of each apple.

- Optional: Sprinkle chopped nuts over the apples.

- Bake for 25–30 minutes, or until the apples are soft.

Nutritional Value:

- Calories: Approximately 180 per serving

- Fiber: 5g

- Vitamin C: 14% of daily recommended intake

Cooking Time: 25-30 minutes

8. Pumpkin Buckwheat Bowl:

Ingredients:

cup buckwheat groats

- cups water
- 1 cup pumpkin puree
- 1/4 cup maple syrup
- 1 teaspoon pumpkin pie spice
- 1/2 cup milk (dairy or plant-based)
- 1/4 cup chopped nuts (for topping) Fresh fruit for garnish (optional)

Preparation:

1. Rinse buckwheat groats under cold water.
2. In a saucepan, combine buckwheat groats and water. Bring to a boil, then reduce heat and simmer for 15-20 minutes, until cooked.
3. In a separate bowl, mix pumpkin puree, maple syrup, and pumpkin pie spice.

4. Stir the pumpkin mixture into the cooked buckwheat.

5. Add milk to achieve desired consistency.

6. Cook for an additional 5 minutes, stirring occasionally.

7. Serve in bowls, topped with chopped nuts and fresh fruit if desired.

Nutritional Value:

- Calories: Approximately 380 per serving

- Protein: 10g

- Fiber: 8g

Cooking Time: 20-25 minutes

9. Zoatmeal bowl

Ingredients:

- 1/2 cup rolled oats

- 1/2 cup grated zucchini

- 1 cup almond milk

- 1 tablespoon chia seeds

- 1 tablespoon maple syrup

- 1/2 teaspoon cinnamon

- 1/4 teaspoon vanilla extract
- Pinch of salt

Preparation:

1. In a saucepan, combine rolled oats, grated zucchini, almond milk, chia seeds, maple syrup, cinnamon, vanilla extract, and a pinch of salt.
2. Cook over medium heat, stirring occasionally, until the mixture thickens and oats are cooked (about 5-7 minutes).
3. Transfer to a bowl and top with your favorite fruits, nuts, or seeds.

Nutritional Value:

- Approx. 350 calories
- Rich in fiber, vitamins, and antioxidants

Cooking Time:

10 minutes

10. Cheesy Tofu Scramble on Avocado Toast

Ingredients:

- 200g firm tofu, crumbled
- tablespoon nutritional yeast
- 1/2 teaspoon turmeric
- 1/4 teaspoon garlic powder
- Salt and pepper to taste
- slices whole grain bread
- 1 ripe avocado, mashed

Preparation:

1. In a skillet, sauté crumbled tofu until slightly browned.
2. Add nutritional yeast, turmeric, garlic powder, salt, and pepper Mix thoroughly and simmer for another 2-3 minutes.
3. Toast the bread slices and spread mashed avocado on top.
4. Spoon the cheesy tofu scramble over the avocado toast.

Cooking Time: 15 minutes

Lunch Recipes

1. Meat & Veggie Roll-ups

Ingredients:

- 1 pound thinly sliced beef or chicken

- 1 zucchini, thinly sliced

- 1 bell pepper, thinly sliced

- 1 tablespoon olive oil Salt and pepper to taste

Preparation:

1. Lay out the meat slices and season with salt and pepper.

2. Place a few slices of zucchini and bell pepper on each meat slice.

3. Roll up the slices and secure with toothpicks.

4. Brush the roll-ups with olive oil.

5. Grill or pan-sear for 5-7 minutes, turning to cook all sides.

Nutritional Value:

- High in protein and vegetables
- Nutrient content depends on specific meat and veggies chosen.

Cooking Time:

15 minutes

2. Strawberry, Cucumber & Feta Salad

Ingredients:

- 2 cups strawberries, sliced
- 1 cucumber, thinly sliced
- 1/2 cup crumbled feta cheese
- 1/4 cup balsamic vinaigrette
- Fresh mint leaves for garnish

Preparation:

1. Combine strawberries, cucumber, and feta in a bowl.
2. Drizzle with balsamic vinaigrette and toss gently.
3. Garnish with fresh mint leaves.

Nutritional Value:

- Low in calories, rich in vitamins and antioxidants.

Cooking Time:

10 minutes (mainly chopping and assembling)

3. Green beans, potatoes and chicken sausage

Ingredients:

- 1 lb green beans, trimmed
- 1 lb baby potatoes, halved
- lb chicken sausage, sliced
- tbsp olive oil
- 1 tsp garlic powder
- 1 tsp onion powder Salt and pepper to taste

Preparation:

1. Preheat oven to 400°F (200°C).
2. In a large bowl, toss green beans, potatoes, and chicken sausage with olive oil, garlic powder, onion powder, salt, and pepper.

3. Spread the mixture evenly on a baking sheet..

4. Roast in the preheated oven for 25-30 minutes or until potatoes are tender and golden brown. Serve hot and enjoy!

Nutritional Value:

- This dish provides a good balance of proteins, fiber, and essential nutrients.

- Green beans are rich in vitamins A and C, as well as fiber.

- Potatoes offer potassium, vitamin C, and B-vitamins.

- Chicken sausage adds protein and flavor.

Cooking Time:

Approximately 25-30 minutes.

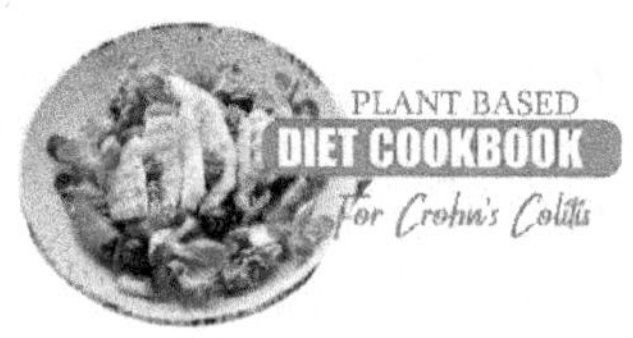

4. Lunch Frittata

Ingredients:

- 6 large eggs
- 1/2 cup milk
- 1 cup diced vegetables (bell peppers, tomatoes, onions)
- 1 cup cooked and diced ham or bacon
- 1 cup shredded cheese
- Salt and pepper to taste 2 tbsp olive oil

Preparation:

1. Preheat oven to 375°F (190°C).
2. In a mixing bowl, combine eggs, milk, salt, and pepper.
3. Heat the olive oil in an oven-safe skillet over medium heat.
4. Saute the vegetables until tender, then add the ham or bacon. Pour the egg mixture into the skillet with the other ingredients.
5. Sprinkle the shredded cheese over top.
6. Cook for 3-4 minutes on the stovetop before transferring the skillet to the preheated oven. Bake for 15-20 minutes,

until the frittata is firm and golden brown. Slice and serve.

Nutritional Value:

- High in protein from eggs and ham/bacon.
- Vegetables contribute vitamins and minerals.
- Cheese provides calcium and additional protein.

Cooking Time:

Approximately 20-25 minutes.

Enjoy your delicious and nutritious meals!

5. Chicken Noodle Soup

Ingredients:

- 1 pound (450g) boneless, skinless chicken breasts
- 8 cups (1.9 liters) chicken broth
- 2 carrots, peeled and sliced
- 2 celery stalks, sliced
- 1 medium onion, chopped
- 3 cloves garlic, minced

- 1 teaspoon dried thyme
- 1 teaspoon dried rosemary
- 8 oz (227g) egg noodles
- Salt and pepper to taste Fresh parsley for garnish

Preparation:

1. In a large pot, bring chicken broth to a simmer.
2. Combine the chicken breasts, carrots, celery, onion, garlic, thyme, and rosemary. Simmer for 20-25 minutes, or until the chicken is thoroughly cooked.
3. Remove chicken, shred it, and return to the pot.
4. Add egg noodles and cook until tender.
5. Season with salt and pepper, garnish with fresh parsley.

Nutritional Value:

- Approximate serving size: 1 cup
- Calories: 200
- Protein: 15g
- Carbohydrates: 20g
- Fat: 6g

Cooking Time:

Total: 40-45 minutes

6. Beet Hummus with Grilled Chicken (or Tofu) Sandwich

Ingredients:

- 1 cup (250g) cooked beets, peeled and diced
- can (15 oz) chickpeas, drained and rinsed
- 1/4 cup (60ml) olive oil
- tablespoons tahini
- 1 clove garlic, minced
- Salt and pepper to taste
- Sliced grilled chicken or tofu
- Whole grain bread
- Fresh spinach leaves
- Optional: Sliced cucumber, tomato

Preparation:

1. In a food processor, combine beets, chickpeas, olive oil, tahini, and garlic. Blend until smooth. Season with salt and pepper to taste.
2. Toast whole grain bread slices.
3. Spread beet hummus on one side of each slice.

4. Layer grilled chicken or tofu, spinach, cucumber, and tomato.

5. To make a sandwich, top with an additional slice of bread.

Nutritional Value:

- Approximate serving size: 1 sandwich

- Calories: 400

- Protein: 20g

- Carbohydrates: 45g

- Fat: 18g

Cooking Time:

Total: 20-25 minutes (including grilling time)

7. Miso ramen soup

Ingredients:

- 200g ramen noodles

- 4 cups vegetable broth

- 3 tbsp miso paste

- 1 cup sliced mushrooms

- 1 cup sliced bok choy

- cup tofu, cubed

- cloves garlic, minced

- tbsp ginger, grated

- green onions, chopped

- 1 tbsp soy sauce

- 1 tsp sesame oil

Preparation:

1. Cook ramen noodles according to package instructions.

2. In a pot, bring vegetable broth to a simmer.

3. Dissolve miso paste in a ladle of hot broth, then add it back to the pot.

4. Add mushrooms, bok choy, tofu, garlic, ginger, and simmer for 5-7 minutes.

5. Stir in soy sauce and sesame oil.

6. Serve hot, garnished with green onions.

Nutritional Value:

- Calories: 350 per serving

- Protein: 15g

- Carbohydrates: 50g

- Fat: 10g

- Fiber: 5g

Cooking Time: 20 minutes

8. Butternut Squash & Tofu Soup

Ingredients:

- 1 medium butternut squash, peeled and diced
- 200g firm tofu, cubed
- onion, chopped
- carrots, sliced
- cups vegetable broth 2 cloves garlic, minced
- tsp curry powder
- Salt and pepper to taste
- tbsp olive oil
- Fresh parsley for garnish

Preparation:

1. In a large pot, sauté onion and garlic in olive oil until translucent.

2. Add butternut squash, carrots, and curry powder; cook for 5 minutes.

3. Pour in vegetable broth and bring to a boil, then simmer until veggies are tender.

4. Add the tofu chunks and season with salt and pepper.

5. Simmer for an additional 10 minutes.

6. Garnish with fresh parsley before serving.

Nutritional Value:

- Calories: 250 per serving
- Protein: 12g
- Carbohydrates: 30g
- Fat: 12g
- Fiber: 8g

Cooking Time: 30 minutes

9. Butternut squash & tofu soup

Ingredients:

- 1 medium butternut squash, peeled and diced
- 200g firm tofu, cubed
- onion, finely chopped
- cloves garlic, minced
- 1 carrot, diced
- 1 celery stalk, chopped
- 4 cups vegetable broth
- 1 teaspoon ground ginger
- 1 teaspoon ground cumin
- Salt and pepper to taste 2 tablespoons olive oil

Preparation:

1. In a large pot, heat the olive oil over medium heat.
2. Add the chopped onion and garlic and sauté until fragrant.
3. Add diced butternut squash, carrot, and celery, cook for 5 minutes.
4. Pour in vegetable broth, add ground ginger and cumin, season with salt and pepper.

5. Bring to a boil, then reduce heat and simmer for 20-25 minutes or until vegetables are tender.

6. Add cubed tofu and cook for an additional 5 minutes.

7. Adjust seasoning if needed and serve hot.

Nutritional Value:

- Calories: Approximately 200 per serving

- Protein: 10g

- Carbohydrates: 25g

- Fiber: 5g

- Fat: 8g

Cooking Time: 30-35 minutes

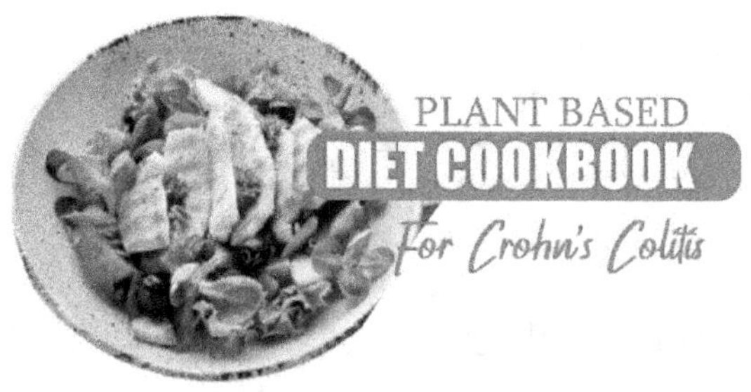

10. Tuna Salad on Toast

Ingredients:

- can (170g) tuna, drained
- tablespoons mayonnaise
- 1 tablespoon Dijon mustard
- 1 celery stalk, finely chopped
- 1/4 red onion, finely diced
- Salt and pepper to taste
- 4 slices whole-grain bread Lettuce leaves for topping

Preparation:

1. In a bowl, mix tuna, mayonnaise, Dijon mustard, chopped celery, and red onion.
2. Season with salt and pepper, adjusting to taste.
3. Toast the whole-grain bread slices.
4. Spoon the tuna salad onto each slice of toast.
5. Topp with lettuce leaves and serve.

Nutritional Value:

- Calories: Approximately 300 per serving
- Protein: 15g

- Carbohydrates: 30g

- Fiber: 5g

- Fat: 15g

Cooking Time: 10 minutes

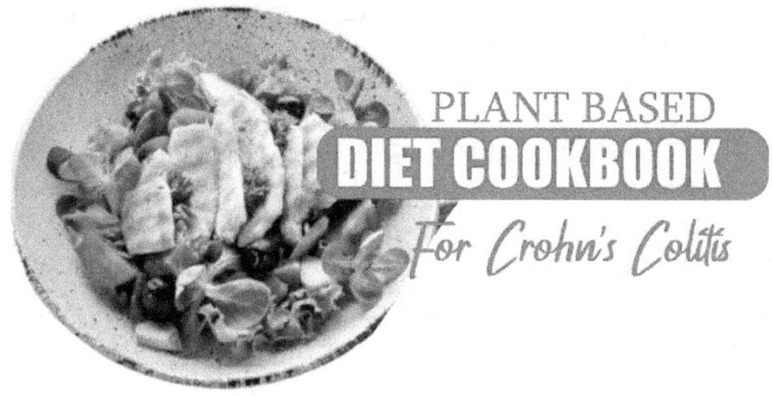

1.Stuffed butternut squash

Ingredients:

- 1 medium-sized butternut squash
- cup quinoa
- cups vegetable broth
- 1 cup black beans (canned and drained)
- 1 cup corn kernels (fresh or frozen)
- 1 red bell pepper, diced
- 1 tablespoon olive oil
- 1 teaspoon cumin
- 1 teaspoon chili powder
- Salt and pepper to taste
- 1/2 cup grated cheddar cheese (optional)

Preparation:

1. Preheat oven to 400°F (200°C).
2. Cut butternut squash in half lengthwise, scoop out seeds, and place on a baking sheet.
3. Roast squash for 30-40 minutes until tender.

4. Meanwhile, rinse quinoa and cook in vegetable broth according to package instructions. In a pan, sauté olive oil, red pepper, corn, and black beans. Add cumin, chili powder, salt, and pepper.

5. Combine cooked quinoa and sautéed vegetables.

6. Stuff the roasted squash halves with the quinoa mixture. Optional: sprinkle with cheddar cheese. Bake for an additional 10 minutes until the cheese melts.

Nutritional Value:

- High in fiber and protein.
- Rich in vitamins A and C.

Approximate cooking time: 1 hour.

2. Buddha Bowl:

Ingredients:

- 1 cup cooked brown rice
- 1 cup chickpeas (canned and rinsed)
- 1 cup broccoli florets
- 1 cup shredded carrots
- cup cherry tomatoes, halved

- 1/2 avocado, sliced

- tablespoons tahini dressing

- 1 tablespoon olive oil

- 1 teaspoon soy sauce Sesame seeds for garnish

Preparation:

1. Steam broccoli florets until tender-crisp.

2. In a pan, sauté chickpeas with olive oil and soy sauce until golden.

3. Assemble the bowl with brown rice, chickpeas, broccoli, carrots, tomatoes, and avocado.

4. Drizzle with tahini dressing and sprinkle sesame seeds on top.

Nutritional Value:

- A balanced combination of carbohydrates, protein, and healthy fats

- Packed with vitamins and minerals.

Approximate cooking time: 30 minutes.

Enjoy your wholesome and nutritious meals!

3. Mediterranean bowl

Ingredients:

- 1 cup cooked quinoa
- 1 cup cherry tomatoes, halved
- cucumber, diced
- 1/2 cup Kalamata olives, pitted and sliced
- 1/2 cup feta cheese, crumbled
- 1/4 cup red onion, finely chopped
- tablespoons olive oil
- 1 tablespoon lemon juice
- 1 teaspoon dried oregano
- Salt and pepper to taste

Preparation:

1. In a large bowl, combine quinoa, cherry tomatoes, cucumber, olives, feta cheese, and red onion.
2. In a small bowl, whisk together olive oil, lemon juice, dried oregano, salt, and pepper. Pour the dressing over the quinoa mixture and toss to incorporate.
3. Serve immediately, or refrigerate for later.

Nutritional Value:

- Calories: Approximately 400 per serving

- Protein: 12g

- Fiber: 8g

- Healthy fats from olive oil and feta.

Cooking Time:

15 minutes (assuming quinoa is pre-cooked).

4. Burrito Bowl

Ingredients:

- 1 cup cooked brown rice

- 1 cup black beans, drained and rinsed

- 1 cup corn kernels (fresh or frozen)

- 1 cup diced bell peppers (assorted colors)

- 1 cup cherry tomatoes, halved

- 1/2 cup shredded cheddar cheese

- 1/4 cup fresh cilantro, chopped

- 1 avocado, sliced

- Salsa and sour cream for topping

Preparation:

- In a bowl, layer brown rice, black beans, corn, bell peppers, cherry tomatoes, cheese, and cilantro.
- Top with avocado slices, salsa, and sour cream.
- Mix everything together before eating to combine flavors.

Nutritional Value:

- Calories: Approximately 450 per serving
- Protein: 14g
- Fiber: 10g
- Healthy fats from avocado.

Cooking Time:

20 minutes (assuming rice and beans are pre-cooked).

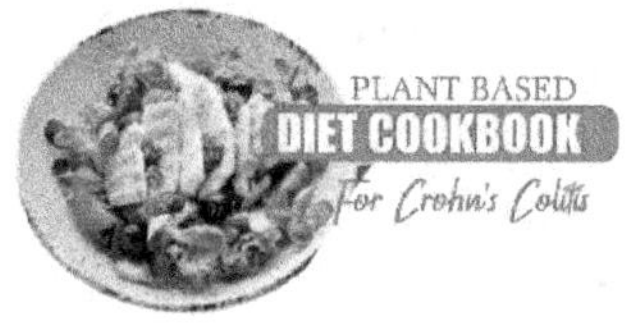

5. Salmon dinner

Ingredients:

- 2 salmon fillets (about 6 oz each)

- 1 tablespoon olive oil

- Salt and pepper to taste

- lemon, sliced

- cloves garlic, minced 1 teaspoon dried dill

Preparation:

1. Preheat the oven to 400°F (200°C).

2. Arrange the salmon fillets on a baking pan lined with parchment paper.

3. Drizzle the fillets with olive oil and season with salt, pepper, chopped garlic, and dried dill.

4. Place lemon slices on top of the fish.

5. Bake for 15-20 minutes, or until the salmon is thoroughly cooked and readily flaked with a fork.

Nutritional Value:

Calories: Approximately 300 per serving

Protein: 25g

Fat: 20g Carbohydrates: 2g

Cooking Time:

15-20 minutes

6. Quinoa and Vegetable Stir-Fry

Ingredients:

- cup quinoa
- cups water or vegetable broth
- 1 tablespoon vegetable oil
- onion, diced
- bell peppers, thinly sliced
- 1 zucchini, diced
- cup broccoli florets
- carrots, julienned
- cloves garlic, minced
- 1/4 cup soy sauce
- 1 tablespoon sesame oil
- 1 tablespoon rice vinegar
- 1 teaspoon ginger, grated

Preparation:

1. Rinse the quinoa under cool water.

2. In a saucepan, mix the quinoa with the water or vegetable broth. Bring to a boil, then reduce heat, cover, and simmer for 15 minutes, or until the quinoa is done.

3. In a large skillet, heat the vegetable oil over medium heat. Sauté onions and garlic until aromatic.

4. Combine bell peppers, zucchini, broccoli, and carrots. Stir-fry the vegetables for 5-7 minutes, until they are soft yet still crisp.

5. Mix in the cooked quinoa, soy sauce, sesame oil, rice vinegar, and shredded ginger. Cook for a another 2-3 minutes, stirring until combined.

Nutritional Value:

- Calories: Approximately 350 per serving

- Protein: 10g

- Fat: 8g

- Carbohydrates: 60g

Cooking Time:

30 minutes

7. Chickpea and Spinach Curry

Ingredients:

- 2 cups chickpeas, cooked
- 4 cups spinach, chopped
- 1 onion, finely chopped
- 3 tomatoes, pureed
- 2 cloves garlic, minced
- 1-inch ginger, grated
- 1 teaspoon cumin seeds
- 1 teaspoon coriander powder
- 1/2 teaspoon turmeric powder
- 1/2 teaspoon chili powder
- teaspoon garam masala
- Salt to taste
- tablespoons cooking oil
- 1 cup water

Preparation:

1. Heat oil in a pan, add cumin seeds, onions, garlic, and ginger. Sauté until onions are golden brown.
2. Add tomato puree, turmeric, coriander powder, chili powder, and salt. Cook until oil separates.
3. Stir in chickpeas and spinach. Add water and cook for 15-20 minutes.
4. Sprinkle garam masala, and cook for an additional 5 minutes.
5. Serve hot, garnished with fresh cilantro.

Nutritional Value:

- Approximate serving size: 1 cup
- Calories: 250
- Protein: 10g
- Fiber: 8g
- Fat: 8g

Cooking Time:

Approximately 30-40 minutes.

8. Zucchini Noodles with Tomato Basil Sauce:

Ingredients:

- 4 medium zucchinis, spiralized
- 2 cups cherry tomatoes, halved
- 2 cloves garlic, minced
- 1/4 cup fresh basil, chopped
- 2 tablespoons olive oil
- Salt and pepper to taste Grated Parmesan cheese (optional)

Preparation:

1. Heat olive oil in a pan, add garlic and sauté until fragrant.
2. Add cherry tomatoes, cook until they start to soften.
3. Toss in zucchini noodles, cook for 3-5 minutes until tender.
4. Stir in basil, salt, and pepper. Cook for an additional 2 minutes.
5. Optional: Sprinkle with Parmesan cheese before serving.

Nutritional Value:

- Approximate serving size: 1.5 cups
- Calories: 120
- Protein: 5g
- Fiber: 4g
- Fat: 8g

Cooking Time:

Approximately 15-20 minutes.

9. Stuffed bell peppers with black beans and quinoa:

Ingredients:

- 4 large bell peppers
- 1 cup quinoa
- 1 can (15 oz) of black beans, drained and rinsed
- 1 cup corn kernels (fresh or frozen)
- 1 cup diced tomatoes
- cup diced onion
- cloves garlic, minced
- 1 teaspoon cumin

- 1 teaspoon chili powder

- 1/2 teaspoon smoked paprika

- Salt and pepper to taste

- 1 cup shredded cheese (optional) Fresh cilantro for garnish

Preparation:

1. Preheat the oven to 375°F (190°C).

2. Cook quinoa according to package instructions.

3. Cut the tops off the bell peppers, remove seeds, and blanch in boiling water for 3-5 minutes. In a large mixing bowl, combine cooked quinoa, black beans, corn, tomatoes, onion, garlic, cumin, chili powder, smoked paprika, salt, and pepper.

4. Stuff each bell pepper with the quinoa mixture and place them in a baking dish.

5. If desired, add shredded cheese over each stuffed pepper.

6. Bake for 25–30 minutes, or until the peppers are soft.

7. Garnish with fresh cilantro before serving.

Nutritional Value:

- Calories: Approximately 300 per stuffed pepper
- Protein: 10g
- Carbohydrates: 50g
- Fat: 6g
- Fiber: 10g

Cooking Time:

Approximately 45-50 minutes

10. Lentil and Vegetable Soup:

Ingredients:

- 1 cup dried green or brown lentils
- onion, diced
- carrots, diced
- celery stalks, diced
- cloves garlic, minced
- 1 can (15 oz) diced tomatoes
- 6 cups vegetable broth
- 1 teaspoon dried thyme

- 1 teaspoon dried oregano
- bay leaf
- Salt and pepper to taste
- cups chopped kale or spinach 2 tablespoons olive oil

Preparation:

1. Rinse lentils under cold water.
2. In a large pot, sauté onion, carrots, celery, and garlic in olive oil until softened.
3. Add lentils, diced tomatoes, vegetable broth, thyme, oregano, bay leaf, salt, and pepper.
4. Bring to a boil, then lower the heat and simmer for 25-30 minutes, or until the lentils are cooked.
5. Cook, stirring in the chopped kale or spinach, until wilted. Before serving, be sure to remove the bay leaf.

Nutritional Value:

Calories: Approximately 250 per serving

Protein: 12g

Carbohydrates: 40g

Fat: 5g

Fiber: 12g   Cooking Time: 45 minutes

Dessert Recipes

1. Pumpkin energy balls

Ingredients:

- 1 cup rolled oats
- 1/2 cup pumpkin puree
- 1/4 cup honey
- 1/2 cup almond butter
- 1/2 cup shredded coconut
- 1 teaspoon pumpkin spice
- 1/2 teaspoon vanilla extract
- A pinch of salt

Preparation:

1. In a bowl, combine rolled oats, pumpkin puree, honey, almond butter, shredded coconut, pumpkin spice, vanilla extract, and a pinch of salt.
2. Mix until well combined.
3. Chill the mixture in the fridge for 30 minutes.
4. Once cold, form the mixture into bite-sized balls. Keep in an airtight jar in the refrigerator.

Nutritional Value:

- Serving Size: 2 balls
- Calories: 150
- Protein: 3g
- Carbohydrates: 18g
- Fat: 8g
- Fiber: 2g

Cooking Time:

30 minutes (including chilling time)

2. Fig Yogurt Bark:

Ingredients:

- 2 cups Greek yogurt
- 1/2 cup chopped figs
- 1/4 cup honey
- 1/4 cup chopped almonds 1 teaspoon vanilla extract

Preparation:

1. In a bowl, mix Greek yogurt, chopped figs, honey, chopped almonds, and vanilla extract.

2. Line a baking sheet with parchment paper.

3. Spread the yogurt mixture evenly across the parchment paper.

4. Freeze for at least 2 hours or until firm.

5. Break the bark into pieces before serving.

Nutritional Value:

- Serving Size: 1/4 cup

- Calories: 80

- Protein: 4g

- Carbohydrates: 10g

- Fat: 3g

- Fiber: 1g

Freezing Time:

2 hours

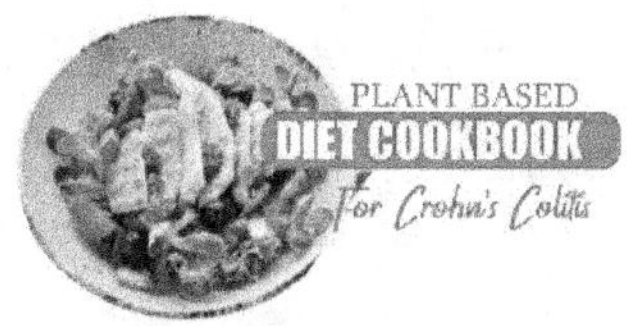

3. Orange Cranberry Muffins

Ingredients:

- 1 ½ cups all-purpose flour
- 1/2 cup sugar
- 1 teaspoon baking powder
- 1/2 teaspoon baking soda
- 1/4 teaspoon salt
- 1/2 cup unsalted butter, melted
- 1/2 cup orange juice
- 1 tablespoon orange zest
- 1 large egg
- 1 cup coarsely chopped fresh or frozen cranberries.

Preparation:

1. Preheat oven to 375°F (190°C).
2. In a large mixing basin, add flour, sugar, baking powder, soda, and salt.
3. In a separate bowl, combine the melted butter, orange juice, zest, and egg.
4. Stir together the wet and dry ingredients until just mixed. Fold in the chopped cranberries.
5. Fill muffin cups about two-thirds full.

6. Bake for 18–20 minutes, or until a toothpick inserted comes out clean. Let the muffins cool for 5 minutes before transferring to a wire rack.

Nutritional Value:

- Calories: 180 per muffin
- Protein: 2g
- Carbohydrates: 26g
- Fat: 8g
- Fiber: 1g

Cooking Time:

18-20 minutes

4. Loaded Chia Pudding

Ingredients:

- 1/4 cup chia seeds
- 1 cup almond milk
- tablespoon maple syrup
- 1/2 teaspoon vanilla extract
- tablespoons Greek yogurt

- 1/2 cup mixed berries
- 1 tablespoon shredded coconut
- 1 tablespoon chopped nuts

Preparation:

1. In a bowl, combine the chia seeds, almond milk, maple syrup, and vanilla extract. Stir well and chill for at least 4 hours, or overnight.
2. Before serving, top chia pudding with Greek yogurt, mixed berries, shredded coconut, and chopped nuts.

Nutritional Value:

Calories: 250 per serving

Protein: 7g

Carbohydrates: 28g

Fat: 13g

Fiber: 10g

5. Apple Pumpkin Bread

Ingredients:

- 2 cups all-purpose flour
- 1 teaspoon baking soda
- 1/2 teaspoon baking powder
- 1/2 teaspoon salt
- 1 teaspoon cinnamon
- 1/2 teaspoon nutmeg
- 1/2 cup unsalted butter, softened
- cup sugar
- large eggs
- 1 cup canned pumpkin puree
- 1 cup grated apple
- 1/2 cup chopped walnuts (optional)

Preparation:

1. Preheat oven to 350°F (175°C).
2. In a bowl, whisk together flour, baking soda, baking powder, salt, cinnamon, and nutmeg. In another bowl,

cream together butter and sugar. Add the eggs one at a time, beating thoroughly after each addition.

3. Stir in pumpkin puree, grated apple, and chopped walnuts.

4. Gradually add dry ingredients to the wet ingredients, mixing until just combined.

5. Pour batter into a greased loaf pan and bake for 55-60 minutes or until a toothpick comes out clean.

Nutritional Value:

- Calories: 220 per slice

- Protein: 4g

- Carbohydrates: 32g

- Fat: 9g

- Fiber: 3g

Cooking Time:

55-60 minutes

BONUS 1

The Paperback of This Version Has A Free 14 Weeks Meal Planner

MY WEEKLY MEAL PLANNER

Date

	Breakfast	Lunch	Dinner
MON			
TUE			
WED			
THU			
FRI			
SAT			
SUN			

SHOPPING LIST:

TO DO LIST

NOTES AND TIPS

24 day sample meal plan.

Day 1:

- Breakfast: Vegan Pancakes with Mixed Berry Yogurt Parfait
- Lunch: Meat & Veggie Roll-ups with Strawberry, Cucumber & Feta Salad
- Dinner: Stuffed Butternut Squash with Quinoa and Vegetable Stir-Fry

Day 2:

- Breakfast: Banana, Blueberry, and Kale Smoothie
- Lunch: Green Beans, Potatoes, and Chicken Sausage with Lunch Frittata
- Dinner: Buddha Bowl

Day 3:

- Breakfast: Overnight Oats with Sliced Banana and Almond Butter
- Lunch: Chicken Noodle Soup with Beet Hummus & Grilled Chicken Sandwich

- Dinner: Mediterranean Bowl

Day 4:

- Breakfast: Eggs, Salmon, and Avocado

- Lunch: Miso Ramen Soup with Tuna Salad on Toast

- Dinner: Burrito Bowl

Day 5

- Breakfast: Zoatmeal Bowl with Fresh Berries

- Lunch: Lentil and Vegetable Soup with Stuffed Bell Peppers

- Dinner: Chickpea and Spinach Curry

Day 6

- Breakfast: "Cheesy" Tofu Scramble on Avocado Toast

- Lunch: Strawberry, Cucumber & Feta Salad with Lunch Frittata

- Dinner: Zucchini Noodles with Tomato Basil Sauce

Day 7

- Breakfast: Banana and Apple Pancakes
- Lunch: Beet Hummus & Grilled Chicken Sandwich with Meat & Veggie Roll-ups
- Dinner: Stuffed Butternut Squash

Day 8

- Breakfast: Yogurt Parfait with Mixed Berries
- Lunch: Green Beans, Potatoes, and Chicken Sausage with Miso Ramen Soup
- Dinner: Buddha Bowl

Day 9

- Breakfast: Overnight Oats with Sliced Banana and Almond Butter
- Lunch: Chicken Noodle Soup with Tuna Salad on Toast
- Dinner: Burrito Bowl

Day 10

- Breakfast: Eggs, Salmon, and Avocado
- Lunch: Butternut Squash & Tofu Soup with Quinoa and Vegetable Stir-Fry
- Dinner: Salmon Dinner

Day 11

- Breakfast: Baked Apple with a sprinkle of cinnamon
- Lunch: Chickpea and Spinach Curry with Zucchini Noodles
- Dinner: Quinoa and Vegetable Stir-Fry

Day 12

- Breakfast: Pumpkin Buckwheat Bowl
- Lunch: Lentil and Vegetable Soup with Stuffed Bell Peppers
- Dinner: Chickpea and Spinach Curry

Day 13

- Breakfast: Zoatmeal Bowl with Fresh Berries
- Lunch: Strawberry, Cucumber & Feta Salad with Lunch Frittata
- Dinner: Zucchini Noodles with Tomato Basil Sauce

Day 14

- Breakfast: Yogurt Parfait with Mixed Berries
- Lunch: Chicken Noodle Soup with Tuna Salad on Toast
- Dinner: Burrito Bowl

Day 15

- Breakfast: Overnight Oats with Sliced Banana and Almond Butter
- Lunch: Butternut Squash & Tofu Soup with Quinoa and Vegetable Stir-Fry
- Dinner: Salmon Dinner

Day 16

- Breakfast: Eggs, Salmon, and Avocado
- Lunch: Chickpea and Spinach Curry with Zucchini Noodles

- Dinner: Quinoa and Vegetable Stir-Fry

Day 17

- Breakfast: Baked Apple with a sprinkle of cinnamon
- Lunch: Lentil and Vegetable Soup with Stuffed Bell Peppers
- Dinner: Chickpea and Spinach Curry

Day 18

- Breakfast: Pumpkin Buckwheat Bowl
- Lunch: Strawberry, Cucumber & Feta Salad with Lunch Frittata
- Dinner: Zucchini Noodles with Tomato Basil Sauce

Day 19

- Breakfast: "Cheesy" Tofu Scramble on Avocado Toast
- Lunch: Beet Hummus & Grilled Chicken Sandwich with Meat & Veggie Roll-ups
- Dinner: Stuffed Butternut Squash

Day 20

- Breakfast: Banana and Apple Pancakes
- Lunch: Green Beans, Potatoes, and Chicken Sausage with Miso Ramen Soup
- Dinner: Buddha Bowl

Day 21

- Breakfast: Yogurt Parfait with Mixed Berries
- Lunch: Chicken Noodle Soup with Tuna Salad on Toast
- Dinner: Burrito Bowl

Day 22

- Breakfast: Overnight Oats with Sliced Banana and Almond Butter
- Lunch: Butternut Squash & Tofu Soup with Quinoa and Vegetable Stir-Fry
- Dinner: Salmon Dinner

Day 23

- Breakfast: Zoatmeal Bowl with Fresh Berries
- Lunch: Strawberry, Cucumber & Feta Salad with Lunch Frittata
- Dinner: Zucchini Noodles with Tomato Basil Sauce

Day 24

- Breakfast: "Cheesy" Tofu Scramble on Avocado Toast
- Lunch: Beet Hummus & Grilled Chicken Sandwich with Meat & Veggie Roll-ups
- Dinner: Stuffed Butternut Squash

Congratulations on completing the 30-day meal plan! Remember to stay hydrated and listen to your body's needs. Feel free to repeat or modify the plan based on your preferences and nutritional goals. Enjoy your delicious and nourishing meals!

Conclusion

You've started a journey of nourishment and healing with this plant-based diet cookbook for Crohn's and colitis. By using vivid, nutrient-dense ingredients, you've not only discovered great dishes, but also provided your body with skills to manage these difficult conditions.

As you relish each dish, keep in mind that you are creating a robust and thriving lifestyle, not just a meal. May the delicacies in these pages nourish your health and inspire you to pursue a healthy lifestyle. Here's to a future in which the combination of nutritious plant-based foods and good health becomes your everyday recipe for energy.

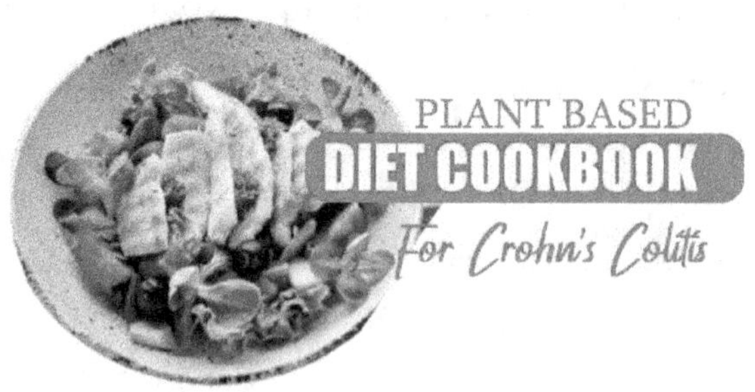

Thank you for looking into our plant-based diet cookbook for Crohn's and colitis. Your dedication to discovering nourishing meals is consistent with our aim of empowering people on their health journeys. Embracing these plant-based meals not only promotes digestive health but also has a favorable environmental impact. Your commitment to comprehensive well-being is very admirable. May these recipes provide you with both culinary delight and health advantages. We appreciate your trust in our cookbook and wish you a delicious and nutritious culinary trip. Thank you for joining our community dedicated to wellness via mindful nutrition.

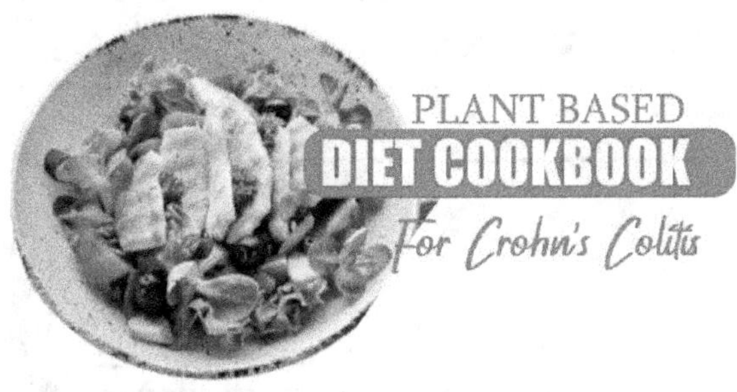

MY WEEKLY MEAL PLANNER

Date

	Breakfast	Lunch	Dinner
MON			
TUE			
WED			
THU			
FRI			
SAT			
SUN			

SHOPPING LIST:

TO DO LIST

NOTES
AND TIPS

MY WEEKLY MEAL PLANNER

Date

	Breakfast	Lunch	Dinner
MON			
TUE			
WED			
THU			
FRI			
SAT			
SUN			

SHOPPING LIST:

To Do List

-
-
-
-

NOTES
AND TIPS

MY WEEKLY MEAL PLANNER

Date

	Breakfast	Lunch	Dinner
MON			
TUE			
WED			
THU			
FRI			
SAT			
SUN			

SHOPPING LIST:

To Do List

NOTES
AND TIPS

MY WEEKLY MEAL PLANNER

Date

	Breakfast	Lunch	Dinner
Mon			
Tue			
Wed			
Thu			
Fri			
Sat			
Sun			

SHOPPING LIST:

-
-
-
-

To Do List

Notes and Tips

MY WEEKLY MEAL PLANNER

Date

	Breakfast	Lunch	Dinner
Mon			
Tue			
Wed			
Thu			
Fri			
Sat			
Sun			

SHOPPING LIST:

To Do List

- ●
- ●
- ●
- ●

Notes And Tips

MY WEEKLY MEAL PLANNER

Date

	Breakfast	Lunch	Dinner
MON			
TUE			
WED			
THU			
FRI			
SAT			
SUN			

SHOPPING LIST:

To Do List

NOTES
AND TIPS

MY WEEKLY MEAL PLANNER

Date

	Breakfast	Lunch	Dinner
MON			
TUE			
WED			
THU			
FRI			
SAT			
SUN			

SHOPPING LIST:

To Do List

- ●
- ●
- ●
- ●

NOTES AND TIPS

MY WEEKLY MEAL PLANNER

Date

	Breakfast	Lunch	Dinner
MON			
TUE			
WED			
THU			
FRI			
SAT			
SUN			

SHOPPING LIST:

To Do List

NOTES
AND TIPS

MY WEEKLY MEAL PLANNER

Date

	Breakfast	Lunch	Dinner
MON			
TUE			
WED			
THU			
FRI			
SAT			
SUN			

SHOPPING LIST:

To Do List

- • ....
- • ....
- • ....
- • ....

NOTES
AND TIPS

MY WEEKLY MEAL PLANNER

Date

	Breakfast	Lunch	Dinner
MON			
TUE			
WED			
THU			
FRI			
SAT			
SUN			

SHOPPING LIST:

To Do List

- ● . . . .
- ● . . . .
- ● . . . .
- ● . . . .

NOTES
AND TIPS

MY WEEKLY MEAL PLANNER

Date

	Breakfast	Lunch	Dinner
MON			
TUE			
WED			
THU			
FRI			
SAT			
SUN			

SHOPPING LIST:

TO DO LIST

NOTES AND TIPS

MY WEEKLY MEAL PLANNER

Date

	Breakfast	Lunch	Dinner
MON			
TUE			
WED			
THU			
FRI			
SAT			
SUN			

SHOPPING LIST:

TO DO LIST

NOTES
AND TIPS

MY WEEKLY MEAL PLANNER

Date

	Breakfast	Lunch	Dinner
Mon			
Tue			
Wed			
Thu			
Fri			
Sat			
Sun			

SHOPPING LIST:

To Do List

-
-
-
-

Notes
And Tips

MY WEEKLY MEAL PLANNER

Date

	Breakfast	Lunch	Dinner
MON			
TUE			
WED			
THU			
FRI			
SAT			
SUN			

SHOPPING LIST:

To Do List

NOTES
AND TIPS

MY WEEKLY MEAL PLANNER

Date

	Breakfast	Lunch	Dinner
MON			
TUE			
WED			
THU			
FRI			
SAT			
SUN			

SHOPPING LIST:

To Do List

NOTES AND TIPS